# TL;DR: fitness
Stefan Cvetkovski

# Table of contents

Disclaimer.................................................................1
Q&A........................................................................2
Chapter 1 – The Food.........................................7
Chapter 2 – The Body.......................................17
Chapter 3 – The Workout.................................24
Chapter 4 – The Supplements.........................33
Chapter 5 – The Mindset..................................35
Chapter 6 – The Start.......................................38
Chapter 7 – The End.........................................40

# Disclaimer

This guide is based on my personal experience and the legitimate research I've encountered over the course of a decade of mental and physical refinement. It covers only the very basics and doesn't delve into molecular biology or the complex biomechanics of the human body. Even though the science holds up and you can easily fact-check it yourself, try to take everything written here with a grain of salt.

**This is NOT an 'easy shortcut' or a 'best way' to approach workouts and dieting.**
One man's 'best way', is another man's journey through hell. It is important to find something that works for you personally.

**This is NOT a detailed program you can follow.**
Think of this as a compact set of rules—a foundation for further improvement. I won't give you any fish, but I can teach you how to recognize quality fish markets.

**This is NOT written by a medical professional.**
I am not liable for any injuries. Consult your physician before performing any vigorous physical activity or caloric restriction. It's all fun and games until a leg stretch kills you or you starve yourself to death by accident.

# Q&A

**What does being fit do for me?**
Basically, it optimizes every aspect of your existence. Some people like lists, so I made a short one:

- It combats a ton of cardiovascular health problems.
- It reduces stress, increases energy levels, improves mental clarity, elevates mood.
- It promotes a positive attitude, discipline and responsibility.
- It fosters a curiosity towards human anatomy, gastronomy, psychology, and you get to know your limits a little better.

**I want those things, are there any downsides?**
There are a couple of side effects people don't tend to mention:

- You might become pretentious and annoying, prancing around with your new healthy obsession.
- You might be perceived as a one-dimensional health freak and a killjoy by your imprudent peers.
- You might start flexing and touching your muscles in public and stare at every reflective surface.
- You might start treating food as numbers and never stop counting calories.

**What if I'm old or obese?**
Same rules apply, with a stronger emphasis on the 'consult a physician' part.

**What if I'm a girl?**
I never said it was boys only. Genders are mostly irrelevant. It will work for all humans.

**What If I'm twelve?**
Finish your homework and consult your legal guardians.

**What if I don't have the time?**
Workouts can last anywhere from 30 minutes to 2-3 hours. If you can't spare at least half an hour you should reconsider your life choices.

**What if I'm a vegetarian, vegan or a level 90 anarchovegan shaman?**
The physical routine will still work, although you will have a tougher time with the nutrition since you don't live by the omnivore's creed.

**Why are you such a condescending prick?**
Trying to be funny here, don't be so easily offended.

**There's a ton of quality books out there, why read your tiny leaflet?**
Because if you can't explain it simply, you don't understand it well enough.

**Will I get huge?**
You don't need big muscles to be healthy and fit. Try to avoid lifting more than 10 times your bodyweight on your first few days and you'll be fine.

**Are YOU huge?**
No. I prefer an easily maintainable physique with a flexible diet.

**That's a poor excuse. Do you even lift?**
Yes, but I have a wide variety of other interests that I can't afford to neglect.

**Can't I just google this info?**
Most of it you can, but it would be redundant. I've been researching and testing stuff on myself for a long time so that you don't have to repeat the process and offend me like this in front of my other readers.

**Why change though? Am I not beautiful and perfect the way I am?**
You can always improve.

A lot of people tend to accept the way they look without really feeling good about themselves. On one hand you should eat whatever you want and look like you want to look, but on the other hand most people think you should look like that person on the cover of that magazine.

**So should I conform to society's standards and listen to other people or just be me?**
It doesn't really matter whether you're mainstream media's poster child or the polar opposite, as long as it's an informed personal decision, and not a justification due to the lack of willpower to improve.

You should also make sure that you're not harming yourself by being overly skinny or obese, unless you're into that whole masochism thing, in which case it's fine and also kinky. ;)

**What about inside beauty, isn't that what really matters?**
Your body speaks volumes even before your words and expressions are taken into consideration. It's a manifestation of your physical well-being and your general lifestyle.

People will make assumptions based on your physical appearance, and in order to withstand their judgment and not be offended or intimidated by a gaze, you need to be comfortable with the state of your body.

**What is love?**
...Unfortunately the Q&A ends here.

If you're really content with every aspect of your existence you should congratulate yourself and wonder why you bought such a book in the first place. If that's not the case, let's move on to the actual content.

# The Food

Food is a fuel packed with delicious nutrients and energy known as calories. Contrary to popular belief, calories are not little harmful gnomes that live in your food. They are simply a unit of measurement used to determine the available energy you would receive from ingesting that certain food item.

Different food offers different amounts of energy, but basically anything can make you fat when taken in excess. **Yes, even fruits and veggies.**

There are three basic types of nutrients known as **macronutrients** that contain the actual energy. In order of my preference they are:

- Fats
- Protein
- Carbohydrates

**Fats** have a bad reputation, but you shouldn't be afraid of them. They are required for hormone production, absorbing vitamins as well as providing the food we eat with a bit of taste, texture and consistency. Fats also supply you with around 9 calories per gram, which is more than double the energy you would get from protein and carbs.

Most of my favorite meals are full of this marvelous and diverse macronutrient. And by diverse, I mean the 3 varieties it comes in:

- Saturated
- Unsaturated
- Trans

**Saturated** fat is often misplaced in the unhealthy fat category due to outdated and faulty studies. This doesn't mean that you should stuff your face with hotdogs and pepperoni. Those overly processed little taste bud ticklers misrepresent saturated fat and everything it stands for. Instead, you should look into some good cuts of meat, eggs and maybe some butter.

**Unsaturated** fat is the hero of the fat bunch. It is represented by nuts, fish and most oils, but if you would like to further complicate things, split it into:

- Monounsaturated
- Polyunsaturated
  - Omega-3
  - Omega-6

**Monounsaturated fat** is present in most types of nuts like almonds, peanuts, cashews and hazelnuts, avocados, olive oil, sunflower oil and a bunch of other healthy stuff.

**Omega 3** and **6** are polyunsaturated essential fatty acids which means you need to ingest them because you can't synthesize them on your own. Research says they offer some nice cardiovascular benefits.

- **Omega-3**s are found in fish, walnuts and oils like canola and flax seed.
- **Omega-6**s are found in olive oil, sunflower oil, most nuts and pumpkin seeds.

There's also Omega-9s and 7s but they don't deserve the attention.

**Trans fat** is the biggest villain of the macros. Stay away from it until further research shows otherwise. Trans fat is strongly correlated to obesity and heart disease, so if you don't want your heart to choke in your own body fat, steer clear from those donuts and french fries unless it's a cheat day.

**Protein** is arguably the most essential macronutrient. You need protein to create, grow, and maintain almost everything. Protein provides you with 4 calories per gram and is made up of smaller building blocks known as amino acids. They can be classified in many groups, but for clarity we'll stick to:

- Essential
- Non-essential

**Essential amino acids**, similar to essential fatty acids must come from ingestion. The nine essential amino acids are:

- Histidine
- Lysine
- Methionine
- Phenylalanine
- Threonine
- Tryptophan
- Isoleucine
- Leucine
- Valine

Isoleucine, Leucine and Valine are known as **BCAAs** or branched-chain amino and are important to remember because unlike the rest of the essentials, these are metabolized and stored primarily in the muscles. They play a crucial role in muscle growth, energy, prevention of muscle breakdown and they also aid the recovery process.

**Nonessential amino acids** are the ones the body can produce even if you don't get them from food. In no particular order they are:

- Alanine
- Asparagine
- Aspartic acid
- Glutamic acid
- Arginine
- Cysteine
- Glutamine
- Tyrosine
- Glycine
- Ornithine
- Proline
- Serine

It's a long list for a basic guide, but it could have been longer if I had explained the roles of every single amino acid. If you're getting your protein from complete sources like meat, eggs or protein supplements,  you won't need to keep track of these pesky aminos.

If you're vegan, vegetarian, spoiled or picky however, you might need to combine different food items in order to taste the whole rainbow.[*]


**Carbohydrates** are basically sugars. They contain 4 calories per gram and are split into monosaccharides, disaccharides, oligosaccharides and polysaccharides, which we can further split into glucose, sucrose, maltose, dextrose, fructose, lactose... But enough sweet talk, let's just refer to them as:

- Simple
- Complex

**Simple** carbs are found in bad stuff like refined bread, sugary drinks and candy, although some redeeming nutritional qualities can be found in milk and fruits. Simple carbs are an excellent instant energy source and are practically useless if you are sedentary.

---

[*]There is no such thing as an amino rainbow, only acids.

**Complex** carbs are the ones you should consume if you decide to include carbs in your diet. Complex carbs provide a steady source of energy and are quite satiating. Some nice sources of complex carbs are wholegrain bread, brown rice and green vegetables.

- **Fiber** can be considered a complex carb, but unlike regular sugars, we can't really digest it. It goes through our gut pushing stuff around, promoting healthy gut bacteria and digestion. Fiber can be further split into **soluble** and **insoluble**, but we don't need to make another list as long as you eat your veggies.

**Alcohol**, while not considered a nutrient, contains around 7 calories per gram which is far from a negligible amount. It's basically a poison that messes up your hormones and nutrient absorption. Some occasions may call for a couple of drinks but the cons heavily outweigh the pros. That being said, I love getting utterly wasted every now and then.

**Micronutrients**, also known as **vitamins** and **minerals**, are chemical compounds required in very tiny amounts. Vitamins look like this:

- Vitamin A
- Vitamin B
  - B1
  - B2
  - B3
  - B5
  - B6
  - B7
  - B9
  - B12
- Vitamin C
- Vitamin D*
- Vitamin E
- Vitamin K

---

*Oh don't be so childish.

The minerals can be tricky since there's a lot of debate on which ones are really essential. We'll just stick to:

- Calcium
- Chromium
- Copper
- Fluoride
- Iodine
- Iron
- Magnesium
- Manganese
- Molybdenum
- Phosphorus
- Potassium
- Selenium
- Zinc

Just like the aminos, there is not much to say here without complicating things.

Most of your deficiencies can be covered by **nutrient-dense** foods such as fruits, vegetables, whole grains and meat, so that you don't have to remember how to spell molybdenum or know that it combines with sulfite oxidase to catalyze sulfur-containing amino acids.

Unlike nutrient-dense foods, **empty-calorie** foods or **energy-dense** foods are nutritionally poor food choices, as they contain more calories than nutrients. If you're fat, blame it on cookies, cake, pastries, chips and the rest of the heavily processed long shelf life foods. Not only do they pack a lot of calories, but they also leave you feeling hungry even after you eat something that serves 5 adults.

**Water** is also important but you don't need to monitor your intake. Drink until your pee gets clear and stay away from sodas, soft drinks and fancy coffee.

| | |
|---|---|
| Top tier | Lean meat<br>Vegetables<br>Legumes<br>Eggs |
| Good tier | Nuts<br>Fruits<br>Whole grains<br>Dairy |
| Consider starving | |
| Junk tier | Refined grains<br>Processed meat<br>Sweets and candy |

# The Body

Your body is an efficient machine that breaks down food into energy in order to maintain, repair and build the many aspects of your unholy existence. The distribution of mass may vary, but your body composition always comes down to:

- **Fat free mass** (The organ systems)
  - Cardiovascular
  - Lymphatic
  - Respiratory
  - Digestive
  - Excretory
  - Endocrine
  - Immune
  - Integumentary
  - Nervous
  - Skeletal
  - Muscular
  - Reproductive
  - Urinary
- **Fat mass**
  - Essential body fat
  - Storage body fat

**The fat free mass** is represented by a bunch of organ systems that work in mutual symbiosis. Their performance is greatly determined by your physical activity and diet, and messing up just one of these intricate systems can have a negative effect on all of them. Here's a brief explanation of their jobs:

**The cardiovascular system** transports blood and nutrients to all the cells in your body.

**The lymphatic system** is sort of like the cardiovascular system except it transports a fluid called lymph and it helps the immune system.

**The respiratory system** deals mostly with breathing.

**The digestive system** breaks down food in order to make it fit into the bloodstream and fuel you.

**The excretory system** poops out the waste left by the digestive system.

**The endocrine system** sends out hormones that cause significant changes in the way organs work.

**The immune system** is your licensed antivirus.

**The intergumentary system** is your protective casing made of skin, nails and hair.

**The nervous system** is the reason you can read this, sense things and memorize them.

**The skeletal system** is the spooky scary skeleton that supports your weight.

**The muscular system** provides movement and makes you strong and sexy.

**The reproductive system** is responsible for making cute little babies.

**The urinary system** pees the waste from the blood.

Discussing these systems any further goes beyond the scope of basic information, so in order to avoid a slippery slope and a hundred more pages explaining proper urinary etiquette, we'll just skip the details.

**Essential body fat** is a very important type of body fat stored in small amounts in bone marrow, organs, the central nervous system and muscles. Men have around 3-5%, and there's 8-12% in women because of hormones and child bearing stuff. This type of fat is not your enemy.

**Storage body fat** is entirely your fault and doesn't do much. It's basically leftover food stored all around your body in the shape of lumpy, jiggly cells. It covers the muscles, and prevents them from being admired.

Both the fat free mass and the fat mass have a rate of energy expenditure when at rest. This rate is known as **BMR** or basal metabolic rate and contributes around 70% to your total daily energy expenditure or **TDEE.** The muscles, brain, heart, liver and kidneys play the major roles, while the fat, bones, skin, blood and the rest of the tissues are less energy expending.

A pound of muscle expends more energy than a pound of fat and it also occupies less space, looks leaner and improves your athletic performance.

Body fat on the other hand is a risk factor for obesity, diabetes, high blood pressure, heart disease and something you shouldn't be proud of, but it is not the sole indicator of bad health.

**BMI** or body mass index is an inaccurate measurement based on your height and weight. It doesn't take into account the muscle mass, fat mass or overall body composition. **Don't fall for the 'perfect weight for your height' thing.**

That leaves us with two other contributing factors to your TDEE:

- Thermic Effect of Food
- Physical Activity

**The thermic effect of food** is how much energy you expend processing the food and accounts for 10% of your TDEE. Protein burns around 25% of its total calories just to be digested while fat and carbohydrates each burn around 5%.

**Physical activity** is the biggest variable and has the potential of being the biggest component of your TDEE. If you're a lazy slob, it can be as low as 100 calories per day, but extreme training regimens are known to burn upwards of 3000 calories per day.

**Losing fat mass** or **cutting** requires consuming 500-1000 calories less than your TDEE. There are a lot of diets based on meal frequency, timing, size and composition, but **without a caloric deficit, fat loss is impossible.** Even if you ate nothing but candy at a 1000 calorie deficit, you would still lose fat.

You might also lose a tiny bit of muscle when losing fat, but it's nothing to worry about as long as you don't go too far with your deficit and do some sort of strength training.

**Gaining mass** or **bulking** is all about a daily surplus of 500-1000 calories. If you have a really high BMR you should be as sedentary as possible and cram your maw with copious amounts of food, which happens to be my definition of a good time.

- **Fat gain** only requires a surplus of calories, food composition is irrelevant. Getting fat also creates new fat cells that stay with you forever. When you lose that weight the fat cells simply shrink down in size and remain there to haunt you for the rest of your life.

- **Muscle gain** occurs when the caloric surplus is accompanied by sufficient protein and strength training. It's recommended that you consume at least 1 gram of protein per 1 pound of body weight which equates to 1 gram per 0.45 kg of body weight for us metric folks. Muscle gain at maintenance level is possible but quite hard to pull off, and gains at a caloric deficit can also occur in absolute beginners but only for a while.

# The Workout

The world of physical training gets bigger every day. It's hard to keep track of every new fad, but we can simplify things by breaking down every workout to two fundamental components:

- Aerobic metabolism
- Anaerobic metabolism

**Aerobic metabolism** fuels any long duration low or medium intensity physical activities that get your heart pumping at an increased pace. These activities are also known as **cardio** since they aim to improve your blood flow, heart and lung function, endurance and most of the stuff dealing with oxygen and oxygen transportation. Distance running and walking are some boring examples of what these workouts look like. Avoid long sessions of aerobic exercises if your goal is muscle gain.

**Anaerobic metabolism** fuels the brief periods of high intensity training and creates a hormonal environment beneficial to building muscle, improving strength, speed and explosive power.

The details separating anaerobic and aerobic exercises can get pretty technical and science-y since the body alternates between the two metabolisms constantly, but we can still make a solid list of anaerobic exercises:

- Resistance training
  - Bodybuilding
  - Powerlifting
  - Weightlifting
  - Strongman
  - Calisthenics
- Sprinting
- Plyometrics
- Isometrics

Before we get into the different branches of resistance training, we need to take a look at some terminology:

**Compound movements** involve a lot of muscles and are quite similar to how you naturally move. Progression is pretty easy since more muscles are involved in the movement. The squat, bench press and deadlift are good examples of what a compound exercise looks like.

**Isolation movements** isolate a particular joint or muscle group. Bicep curls for example only work the biceps. These are good for muscles that are lagging behind or making sure your abs stand out because they are the most important thing when it comes to being fit and healthy.*

**DOMS** or **delayed onset muscle soreness** is the muscle ache felt after intense workouts. It usually happens 24 hours after the workout but hits pretty hard even after two or three days.

Working the sore muscle has no effect on recovery and will even reduce your pain for a while. Learn to love this pain unless it's gets sharp or pulsating, in which case it's most likely not DOMS and you should get that checked out.

**Reps** or repetitions is how many times you repeat a certain movement.

- **1RM** or one repetition maximum is the maximum weight you can lift for 1 rep.

**Sets** consist of multiple reps.

**Volume** is the amount of sets and reps done during a workout.

---

*They are not. That was sarcasm.

**Intensity** is how hard you push yourself which is relative to your 1RM. The closer you get to your 1RM, the higher the intensity, with 1RM representing 100% intensity.

| Goal | Reps | Intensity |
|------|------|-----------|
| Strength | 1-5 | 85-100% |
| Size | 6-12 | 70-85% |
| Endurance | 13+ | Less than 70% |

**Frequency** is how often you hit a certain muscle group. You have to experiment with this one, because it works differently for each person.

**Flexibility** deals with the length of a muscle and tightness, while **mobility** is about the range of motion of your joints.

**Bodybuilding** is all about size, low body fat and looking good. Strength gains also occur, but they are not the focal point. Bodybuilding incorporates both isolation and compound movements and usually relies on free weights, although machines, bodyweight and elastic bands are not uncommon.

**Powerlifting** is about maximum power and strength. The competitions only care about the bench press, the deadlift and the squat, but other compound movements like barbell rows and shoulder presses are a staple of recreational powerlifting. Since strength is the main focus, body fat isn't an issue. Fat may even prove useful for the lifts and spare more muscle since the body will go for fat instead of muscle when energy is low.

**Weightlifting** or **olympic weightlifting** consists of the snatch and the clean and jerk. While also testing maximum strength, these two movements are more technically difficult than the ones in powerlifting and are significantly more explosive. They also look very pretty and graceful.

**Strongman** is about using strength, endurance and explosive power to pull cars, move rocks and flip tires. Although the training part can be done with some of the regular gym equipment, the contests usually involve pulling actual trucks.

**Calisthenics** or **bodyweight training** is refusing to lift anything but yourself. Using your own body as resistance means it's hard to achieve that 1RM intensity, but there are ways to shake it up. You can slow the movement down, make it explosive or just start using less body parts. An example of progression would be doing one-handed push-ups instead of regular push-ups.

**Sprinting** is jogging on steroids. It's a full body workout at a high intensity, and it offers a metabolic boost that lasts for hours.

**Plyometrics** is jumping in 50 different ways. It's a good way to improve explosiveness and overall performance in sports.

**Isometrics** is working out without moving, but it's not as easy as it sounds. Instead of working with reps, your aim is to hold the position as long as possible. The plank is an example of what a static exercise looks like.

Some activities like recreational sports and martial arts kill two birds with one stone by incorporating both the aerobic and anaerobic metabolism.

We're gonna skip the details on how to play basketball and how to perform the five point palm exploding heart technique.

Instead, we're gonna make a list about:

- Yoga
- Pilates
- Circuit Training
- Interval Training
- Stretching

**Yoga** is about exploring the mind and spiritual enlightenment but it can work wonders as a supplement to any workout. The physical aspect can improve your flexibility and mobility, and meditation can help with relaxation.

**Pilates** is core body work with a ball companion. It mainly focuses on balance and flexibility. It's like a more intense version of yoga without the mental part.

**Circuit training** is a mix of everything. You make a list of exercises, pick the equipment and just cycle through the workout a predetermined number of times until you drop.

**Interval training** is similar to circuit training and alternates between the aerobic and anaerobic systems. An example would be adding a sprint to a steady paced walk every now and then.

- **HIIT** or **High intensity interval training** is working out at maximum intensity followed by shorter periods of rest or low intensity work. Since HIIT relies on extreme intensity, you can do the whole thing in a very short time.

**Stretching** is the act of extending various body parts in order to prevent injuries and improve flexibility and mobility. Always make sure you are flexible enough to perform the full range of motion before doing any type of exercise.

Stretching can be done in a number of ways:

- Ballistic
- Dynamic
- Static
- PNF

**Ballistic stretching** is where you use momentum to force a body part beyond its range of motion. An example is trying to touch your toes while bouncing further every time. Not recommended unless you know what you're doing.

**Dynamic stretching** is swinging body parts in a more controlled manner. Instead of bouncing, you gradually increase the range of motion and the speed of the movement.

**Static stretching** is holding a stretch for at least 30 seconds. Try to avoid static stretching before sprinting or resistance training since it might mess up your performance.

**PNF** stands for proprioceptive neuromuscular facilitation. It's basically static stretching with added contractions and resistance. It's generally better to do it with a partner, but you can also do it solo and blame any injuries on yourself. An example of PNF is someone pushing your leg towards your chest while you're laying on your back.

# THE SUPPLEMENTS

Supplements are exactly what their name implies. They won't do much for someone with poor diet and training. People who are not omnivores benefit greatly from supplements since they often suffer from nutritional deficiencies.

**Protein powders** are a powdered form of the same protein you would otherwise get from food. They aren't harmful at all and you don't need them if you're able to meat* your protein requirements.

**Weight gainers** are protein powders with added carbs and fat. They can often serve as a meal replacement but you shouldn't give up food for them.

**Creatine** provides a boost to strength and muscle size as long as you keep taking it. It's pretty safe and there are no side effects unless you snort it. Don't snort it.

**Multivitamin** and **mineral** supplements are a must if you're on a restrictive diet, but you can take them even if that's not the case.

---

* I am the god of puns. Witness me.

**Caffeine** is like a healthier version of cocaine that boosts your energy levels and revs up your metabolism. You can take it as a pre-workout in supplement form or just drink some coffee, green or black tea. Tolerance is built up quite fast though, and the withdrawal symptoms can be pretty rough.

**Anabolic steroids** are synthetic hormones used to build muscle. They can be extremely dangerous if not used properly and are illegal in most countries.

There's also amino supplements, mixed preworkouts, fat burners and a thing called Ejaculoid, but they're not as relevant.

# THE MINDSET

The mindset is how you approach this whole thing. It can be like exploring a new world, or it can be an improvement of your current one. You're already on a diet and a routine, but you don't see it that way because you probably eat crappy food and your workout consists of occasional walks to the bathroom. If you fit this description and think self-deprecating humor will somehow make up for the bad shape you're in, then I have some tough news for you...

You are not a beautiful or unique snowflake that lives in an alternate world of hedonistic pleasures and mindless self-indulgence, you're just a bad version of a healthy human being. **You are a bad version of yourself**.

When most people realize this and decide to do something about it, they often go for pants-on-head retarded workouts and diets that promise instant results. The rise to the challenge is admirable, but the transition from a commoner to a warrior-philosopher is not an easy one. After a certain point the majority of people fail to perform up to standard and they relapse into the realm where their destructive desires run rampant, while the very few persistent ones manage to adapt and make a long-term commitment to a better life.

It doesn't matter if you failed the first time or the first fifteen times. It doesn't matter how many relapses, new year resolutions and next weeks it takes you to build a habit, as long as you don't stop trying.

By consistently working towards your goal, you will build responsibility, discipline and work ethic. You will have more energy, mental and physical capacity at your disposal to perform whatever pointless and destructive stuff you did before.

But I'm pretty sure you already knew about most of this stuff even before you started reading this book. Every single day the news and social media talk about how a sedentary lifestyle and junk food can kill you. It certainly isn't the lack of information that's stopping you from improving, so what could it be?

Among the many possible psychological and physical reasons you are not on your way to greatness there are two major culprits known as **procrastination** and **cognitive dissonance**.

Whenever you decide to do something productive, and then randomly postpone it because you have more enjoyable things to do, you are procrastinating. The uncomfortable feeling of guilt you experience when you actually realize you're doing something pleasurable instead of doing that important thing you intended is known as cognitive dissonance. You can feel guilty all day and promise yourself that it won't happen again, but the best way to deal with it next time is to act on impulse and **just start it.**

So instead of reading this book and repeat history, you're gonna start being productive right now.

# THE START

This is it, the end of procrastination and the start of a better you. You don't need access to training equipment or food. All you need to do is make a mental note that there is no turning back.

I know it sounds like a big deal but try not to feel intimidated, you're gonna take it step by step.

### Step 1
Tone down the junk

You can either eat smaller portions, eat less frequently, or just quit it altogether. Keep in mind that the more you deprive yourself of your favorite junk food—the more willpower you will need to avoid a relapse.

### Step 2
Amp the nutrition

Keep your protein intake above 100g and fill the rest of it with carbs and fat. Experiment with the ratios and find out what works best for your goals.

### Step 3
Find a workout

Pick your poison and focus on strength, endurance, mobility, speed, aesthetics or try to be a jack of all trades. Aim to hit both the aerobic and anaerobic metabolism.

### Step 4
Stick with it

Sometimes life happens. You need to be able to adapt your program to whatever is thrown at you. There will be days or maybe even weeks where you won't be able to stick to your schedule. Instead of beating yourself up, try to compensate for those lapses.

Stick to these easy steps, and you will be a fit and healthy individual in no time.

| Health and Fitness | |
|---|---|
| Physical aspect | Nutritional aspect |
| ☐ Aerobic exercise<br>☐ Anaerobic exercise<br>☐ Flexibility<br>☐ Mobility | ☐ Healthy fats<br>☐ Complete protein<br>☐ Fiber<br>☐ Micronutrients |

# THE END

It turns out being fit and healthy is not the boring activity that consumes your happiness and prevents you from having fun. It does require hard work, but in the end, the effort should have a positive effect on you and your goals, whatever they may be.

Thank you for taking the time to read a non-native English speaker's largely incoherent booklet.

I wish you the best of luck in achieving the perfect balance of work and play. Try not to tip the scales too much either way.